I0781839

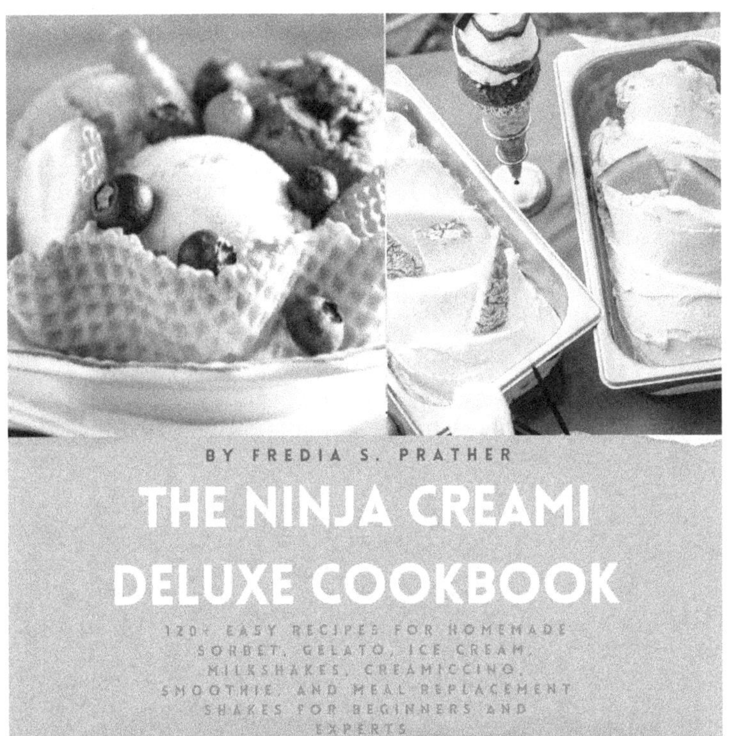

BY FREDIA S. PRATHER
THE NINJA CREAMI
DELUXE COOKBOOK
120+ EASY RECIPES FOR HOMEMADE
SORBET, GELATO, ICE CREAM,
MILKSHAKES, CREAMICCINO,
SMOOTHIE, AND MEAL REPLACEMENT
SHAKES FOR BEGINNERS AND
EXPERTS

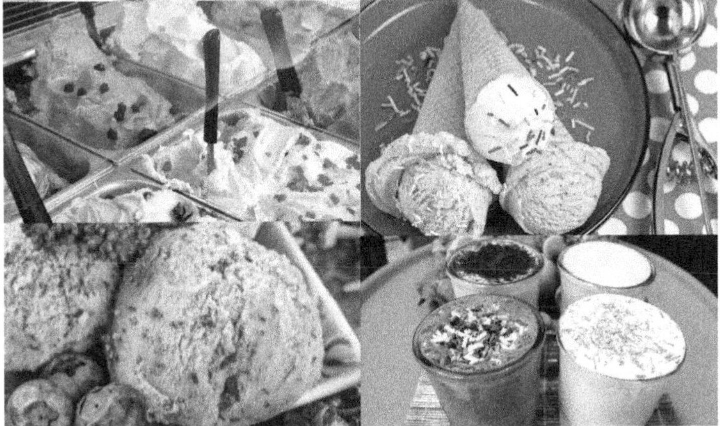

Table of Contents

Introduction

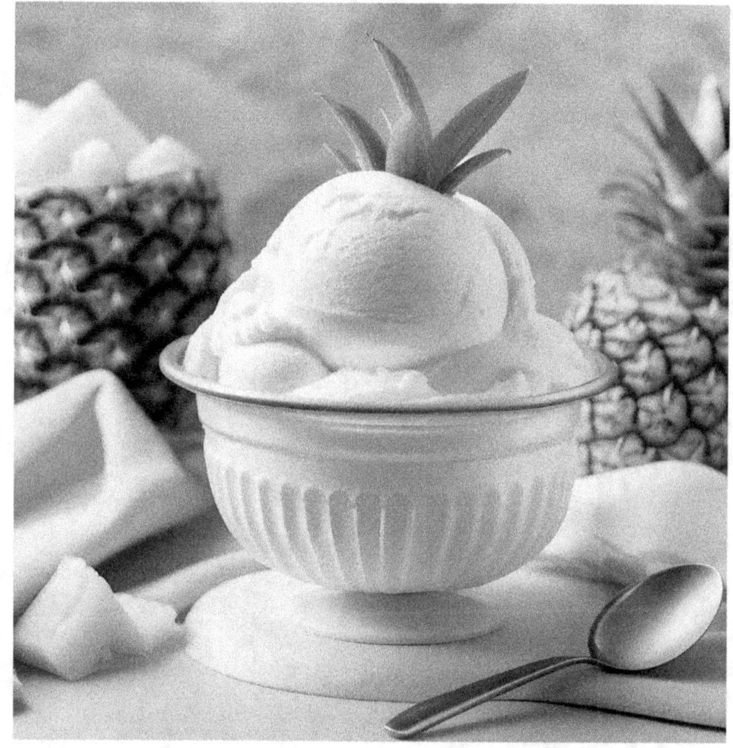

Welcome to "The Ninja Creami Deluxe Cookbook: 120+ Easy Recipes for Homemade Sorbet, Gelato, Ice Cream, Milkshakes, Creamiccino, Smoothie, and Meal Replacement Shakes for Beginners and Experts." This book is your ultimate guide to creating delicious, homemade treats with ease using the versatile Ninja Creami.

Whether you are an expert in the kitchen or just starting your culinary journey, this cookbook is designed to help you make the most of your Ninja Creami. With about 140 recipes, you'll discover a world of flavors and textures that are both delightful and easy to prepare. From refreshing sorbets to indulgent milkshakes, and nutritious smoothies to satisfying meal replacement shakes, there's something for everyone.

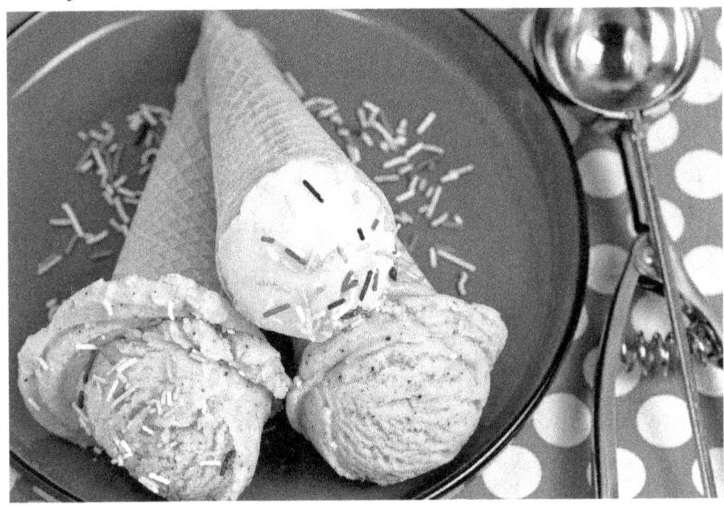

Sorbet

Sorbet is the perfect light and refreshing treat for any time of year. Made with fresh fruits and simple ingredients, our sorbet recipes are a breeze to whip up. Imagine enjoying a tangy lemon sorbet on a hot day or a rich raspberry sorbet for a sophisticated dessert. With the Ninja Creami, you can create these delightful, icy treats in the comfort of your own home.

Ice Cream

Indulge in the creamy, dreamy world of homemade ice cream. Whether you prefer classic flavors like vanilla and chocolate or adventurous options like matcha green tea and salted caramel, our recipes cater to every taste. Using the Ninja Creami, you can achieve that perfect, scoopable texture every time, making every bite a true pleasure.

Gelato

Discover the rich and velvety world of gelato with our easy-to-follow recipes. Gelato, an Italian favorite, is known for its dense and creamy texture, achieved with less air than traditional ice cream. From classic flavors like pistachio and hazelnut to modern twists like tiramisu and lemon basil, our gelato recipes are sure to impress. The Ninja Creami allows you to replicate the authentic taste and texture of gelato right in your kitchen.

Milkshakes

Milkshakes are a beloved favorite, and with our recipes, you can enjoy them in a variety of flavors. From a traditional chocolate milkshake to a tropical pineapple delight, these recipes are sure to satisfy your sweet tooth. The Ninja Creami makes it easy to blend these thick, creamy drinks to perfection.

Creamiccino

For a coffeehouse experience at home, our Creamiccino recipes are a must-try. These frothy, coffee-infused drinks are perfect for a morning pick-me-up or an afternoon treat. With flavors ranging from classic mocha to vanilla caramel, you can enjoy a gourmet coffee experience without leaving your kitchen.

Smoothies

Smoothies are a fantastic way to pack in nutrients while enjoying a delicious treat. Our recipes include a wide range of options, from green detox smoothies to berry-packed blends. Using fresh ingredients and the power of the Ninja Creami, you can create smoothies that are not only tasty but also good for you.

Meal Replacement Shakes

For those busy days when you need a quick and nutritious option, our meal replacement shakes are the perfect solution. These recipes are designed to provide a balanced mix of proteins, carbs, and fats to keep you satisfied and energized. With flavors like peanut butter banana and chocolate almond, you'll look forward to every sip.

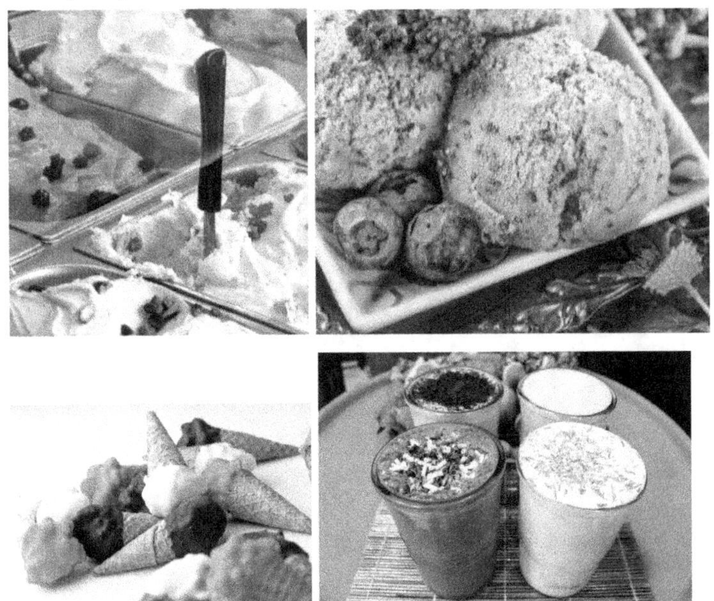

In this cookbook, each recipe is crafted with simple, easy-to-find ingredients and clear instructions, ensuring that you can create mouthwatering treats with confidence. Whether you're making a refreshing sorbet, a creamy ice cream, a thick milkshake, a frothy Creamiccino, a nutritious smoothie, or a satisfying meal replacement shake, the Ninja Creami is your perfect companion.

So, grab your Ninja Creami, gather your ingredients, and let's get started on a delicious adventure. With these easy-to-follow recipes, you'll soon be impressing your family and friends with homemade treats that are as fun to make as they are to eat. Enjoy!

Chapter 1

What You Need To Know About Ninja Creami

The Ninja Creami is a fantastic machine for making homemade frozen treats. It's simple to use and lets you create a variety of delicious desserts with ease. Here are the basics you need to know to get started:

What is the Ninja Creami?

The Ninja Creami is a kitchen appliance designed to make ice cream, gelato, sorbet, milkshakes, and more. It's user-friendly and perfect for anyone who loves homemade desserts.

Key Features:

1. Easy to Use: Just add your ingredients, press a button, and let the machine do the rest.

2. Versatile: It can make a wide range of frozen treats, from creamy ice cream to refreshing sorbets.

3. Customizable: You can experiment with different flavors and ingredients to create your perfect dessert.

Getting Started:

1. Prepare Your Ingredients: Gather the ingredients for your chosen recipe. This might include milk, cream, sugar, fruits, or other flavorings.

2. Mix and Chill: Combine the ingredients as instructed and chill them in the refrigerator for a few hours.

3. Process in the Creami: Once chilled, place the mixture in the Ninja Creami, select the appropriate setting (like ice cream or sorbet), and start the machine.

Basic Recipes:

1. Ice Cream: Mix milk, cream, sugar, and your favorite flavorings (like vanilla or chocolate). Chill, then process in the Creami.

2. Sorbet: Blend fruits with a bit of water and sugar. Chill, then process in the Creami.

3. Milkshakes: Combine ice cream with milk and flavorings. Blend until smooth.

Tips for Success:

1. Use Fresh Ingredients: For the best taste, use fresh and high-quality ingredients.

2. Follow Recipes: Especially when you're starting, follow the recipes closely to get good results.

3. Experiment: Once you're comfortable, try experimenting with new flavors and ingredients.

Cleaning and Maintenance:

1. Easy to Clean: Most parts of the Ninja Creami are dishwasher-safe. After each use, disassemble the machine and clean the parts thoroughly.

2. Regular Maintenance: Regularly check and clean the machine to ensure it continues to work well and lasts a long time.

Why You'll Love the Ninja Creami:

1. Homemade Goodness: Enjoy fresh, homemade ice cream, gelato, and more without any preservatives or artificial ingredients.

2. Fun and Creative: Making your frozen treats is fun and lets you get creative with flavors and ingredients.

3. Convenient: The Ninja Creami makes it easy to whip up delicious desserts whenever you want.

With the Ninja Creami, you can bring the joy of homemade frozen treats into your kitchen. It's easy to use, versatile, and perfect for creating a wide variety of delicious desserts.

Chapter 2

Meal Replacement Shakes Recipes

Here are 20 simple and delicious meal replacement shakes you can make at home. Each recipe includes the ingredients, directions, prep time, cook time, and servings.

1. Banana Oat Shake

Ingredients:

- 1 ripe banana

- 1/2 cup rolled oats

- 1 cup almond milk

- 1 tablespoon peanut butter

- 1 teaspoon honey (optional)

Directions:

- Combine all ingredients in a blender.

- Blend until smooth.

- Pour into a glass and enjoy.

Prep Time: 5 minutes
Cook Time: 0 minutes
Serving: 1

2. Berry Blast Shake

Ingredients:

- 1 cup mixed berries (strawberries, blueberries, raspberries)

- 1 cup Greek yogurt

- 1/2 cup orange juice

- 1 tablespoon honey

Directions:

- Add all ingredients to a blender.

- Blend until smooth.

- Serve immediately.

Prep Time: 5 minutes
Cook Time: 0 minutes
Serving: 1

3. Green Power Shake

Ingredients:

- 1 cup spinach leaves

- 1/2 avocado

- 1 banana

- 1 cup coconut water

- 1 tablespoon chia seeds

Directions:

- Place all ingredients in a blender.

- Blend until smooth.

- Enjoy your green shake.

Prep Time: 5 minutes
Cook Time: 0 minutes
Serving: 1

4. Chocolate Peanut Butter Shake

Ingredients:

- 1 cup milk (dairy or plant-based)

- 1 banana

- 1 tablespoon cocoa powder

- 1 tablespoon peanut butter

- 1 teaspoon honey (optional)

Directions:

- Combine all ingredients in a blender.

- Blend until smooth.

- Pour into a glass and serve.

Prep Time: 5 minutes
Cook Time: 0 minutes
Serving: 1

5. Tropical Mango Shake

Ingredients:

- 1 cup frozen mango chunks

- 1/2 cup pineapple juice

- 1/2 cup Greek yogurt

- 1 tablespoon honey

Directions:

- Add all ingredients to a blender.

- Blend until smooth.

- Serve immediately.

Prep Time: 5 minutes
Cook Time: 0 minutes
Serving: 1

6. Coffee Banana Shake

Ingredients:

- 1 banana

- 1/2 cup brewed coffee (cooled)

- 1/2 cup milk (dairy or plant-based)

- 1 tablespoon oats

- 1 teaspoon vanilla extract

Directions:

- Combine all ingredients in a blender.

- Blend until smooth.

- Pour into a glass and enjoy.

Prep Time: 5 minutes

Cook Time: 0 minutes

Serving: 1

7. Almond Berry Shake

Ingredients:

- 1 cup mixed berries

- 1 cup almond milk

- 1 tablespoon almond butter

- 1 tablespoon honey

Directions:

- Place all ingredients in a blender.

- Blend until smooth.

- Serve immediately.

Prep Time: 5 minutes
Cook Time: 0 minutes
Serving: 1

8. Vanilla Chia Shake

Ingredients:

- 1 cup milk (dairy or plant-based)

- 1 tablespoon chia seeds

- 1 tablespoon vanilla protein powder

- 1 teaspoon honey

Directions:

- Combine all ingredients in a blender.

- Blend until smooth.

- Pour into a glass and enjoy.

Prep Time: 5 minutes
Cook Time: 0 minutes
Serving: 1

9. Peach Smoothie Shake

Ingredients:

- 1 cup frozen peaches

- 1 cup Greek yogurt

- 1/2 cup orange juice

- 1 tablespoon honey

Directions:

- Add all ingredients to a blender.

- Blend until smooth.

- Serve immediately.

Prep Time: 5 minutes
Cook Time: 0 minutes
Serving: 1

10. Coconut Pineapple Shake

Ingredients:

- 1 cup pineapple chunks

- 1/2 cup coconut milk

- 1/2 cup Greek yogurt

- 1 tablespoon honey

Directions:

- Place all ingredients in a blender.

- Blend until smooth.

- Enjoy your tropical shake.

Prep Time: 5 minutes
Cook Time: 0 minutes
Serving: 1

11. Strawberry Banana Shake

Ingredients:

- 1 banana

- 1 cup strawberries

- 1 cup milk (dairy or plant-based)

- 1 tablespoon honey

Directions:

- Combine all ingredients in a blender.

- Blend until smooth.

- Pour into a glass and serve.

Prep Time: 5 minutes
Cook Time: 0 minutes
Serving: 1

12. Blueberry Almond Shake

Ingredients:

- 1 cup blueberries

- 1 cup almond milk

- 1 tablespoon almond butter

- 1 tablespoon honey

Directions:

- Add all ingredients to a blender.

- Blend until smooth.

- Serve immediately.

Prep Time: 5 minutes
Cook Time: 0 minutes
Serving: 1

13. Apple Cinnamon Shake

Ingredients:

- 1 apple, cored and chopped

- 1 cup Greek yogurt

- 1/2 cup milk (dairy or plant-based)

- 1/2 teaspoon cinnamon

- 1 tablespoon honey

Directions:

- Place all ingredients in a blender.

- Blend until smooth.

- Enjoy your shake.

Prep Time: 5 minutes//Cook Time: 0 minutes//Serving: 1

14. Pumpkin Spice Shake

Ingredients:

- 1/2 cup pumpkin puree

- 1 banana

- 1 cup almond milk

- 1/2 teaspoon pumpkin pie spice

- 1 tablespoon honey

Directions:

- Combine all ingredients in a blender.

- Blend until smooth.

- Pour into a glass and serve.

Prep Time: 5 minutes//Cook Time: 0 minutes// Serving: 1

15. Mango Avocado Shake

Ingredients:

- 1 cup frozen mango chunks

- 1/2 avocado

- 1 cup coconut water

- 1 tablespoon honey

Directions:

- Add all ingredients to a blender.

- Blend until smooth.

- Serve immediately.

Prep Time: 5 minutes
Cook Time: 0 minutes
Serving: 1

16. Kiwi Spinach Shake

Ingredients:

- 1 kiwi, peeled and chopped

- 1 cup spinach leaves

- 1 banana

- 1 cup water

- 1 tablespoon honey

Directions:

- Place all ingredients in a blender.

- Blend until smooth.

- Enjoy your green shake.

Prep Time: 5 minutes//Cook Time: 0 minutes//Serving: 1

17. Berry Beet Shake

Ingredients:

- 1 small cooked beet, chopped

- 1 cup mixed berries

- 1 cup Greek yogurt

- 1 tablespoon honey

Directions:

- Combine all ingredients in a blender.

- Blend until smooth.

- Pour into a glass and serve.

Prep Time: 5 minutes
Cook Time: 0 minutes
Serving: 1

18. Coconut Berry Shake

Ingredients:

- 1 cup

- mixed berries

- 1 cup coconut milk

- 1 tablespoon chia seeds

- 1 tablespoon honey

Directions:

- Add all ingredients to a blender.

- Blend until smooth.

- Serve immediately.

Prep Time: 5 minutes
Serving: 1

19. Avocado Kale Shake

Ingredients:

- 1/2 avocado

- 1 cup kale leaves

- 1 banana

- 1 cup almond milk

- 1 tablespoon honey

Directions:

- Place all ingredients in a blender.

- Blend until smooth.

- Enjoy your healthy shake.

Prep Time: 5 minutes
Serving: 1

20. Cinnamon Roll Shake

Ingredients:

- 1 banana

- 1/2 teaspoon cinnamon

- 1 cup Greek yogurt

- 1 cup almond milk

- 1 tablespoon honey

Directions:

- Combine all ingredients in a blender.

- Blend until smooth.

- Pour into a glass and serve.

Prep Time: 5 minutes
Serving: 1

These 20 meal replacement shakes are quick and easy to make, providing you with nutritious and delicious options for any time of the day. Enjoy experimenting with different flavors and ingredients to find your favorites!

Chapter 3

Ice Cream Recipes

Here are 20 delightful ice cream recipes for you to enjoy:

1. Classic Vanilla Ice Cream

Ingredients:

- 2 cups heavy cream

- 1 cup whole milk

- 3/4 cup sugar

- 1 tbsp vanilla extract

Directions:

- In a bowl, mix heavy cream, milk, sugar, and vanilla extract.

- Pour the mixture into an ice cream maker and churn according to the manufacturer's instructions.

- Transfer to a container and freeze for at least 2 hours before serving.

Prep Time: 10 minutes
Cook Time: 20 minutes (churning)
Servings: 4

2. Chocolate Ice Cream

Ingredients:

- 2 cups heavy cream

- 1 cup whole milk

- 3/4 cup sugar

- 1/2 cup cocoa powder

- 1 tsp vanilla extract

Directions:

- In a saucepan, heat milk, sugar, and cocoa powder over medium heat until sugar dissolves.

- Remove from heat and stir in heavy cream and vanilla extract.

- Chill the mixture in the refrigerator for 2 hours.

- Pour into an ice cream maker and churn as per instructions.

- Freeze for 2 hours before serving.

Prep Time: 15 minutes
Cook Time: 20 minutes (churning)
Servings: 4

3. Strawberry Ice Cream

Ingredients:

- 2 cups fresh strawberries, hulled and sliced

- 2 cups heavy cream

- 1 cup whole milk

- 3/4 cup sugar

- 1 tsp lemon juice

Directions:

- Blend strawberries with lemon juice and sugar until smooth.

- In a bowl, mix heavy cream and milk.

- Stir in the strawberry puree.

- Pour into an ice cream maker and churn as per instructions.

- Freeze for 2 hours before serving.

Prep Time: 15 minutes
Cook Time: 20 minutes (churning)
Servings: 4

4. Mint Chocolate Chip Ice Cream

Ingredients:

- 2 cups heavy cream

- 1 cup whole milk

- 3/4 cup sugar

- 1 tsp peppermint extract

- 1 cup chocolate chips

- A few drops of green food coloring (optional)

Directions:

- In a bowl, mix heavy cream, milk, sugar, and peppermint extract.

- Add food coloring if desired.

- Pour into an ice cream maker and churn as per instructions.

- Add chocolate chips in the last 5 minutes of churning.

- Freeze for 2 hours before serving.

Prep Time: 10 minutes
Cook Time: 20 minutes (churning)
Servings: 4

5. Cookies and Cream Ice Cream

Ingredients:

- 2 cups heavy cream

- 1 cup whole milk

- 3/4 cup sugar

- 1 tsp vanilla extract

- 15 crushed Oreo cookies

Directions:

- In a bowl, mix heavy cream, milk, sugar, and vanilla extract.

- Pour into an ice cream maker and churn as per instructions.

- Add crushed Oreos in the last 5 minutes of churning.

- Freeze for 2 hours before serving.

Prep Time: 10 minutes
Cook Time: 20 minutes (churning)
Servings: 4

6. Salted Caramel Ice Cream

Ingredients:

- 2 cups heavy cream

- 1 cup whole milk

- 3/4 cup sugar

- 1/2 cup caramel sauce

- 1/2 tsp sea salt

Directions:

- In a bowl, mix heavy cream, milk, sugar, and caramel sauce.

- Stir in sea salt.

- Pour into an ice cream maker and churn as per instructions.

- Freeze for 2 hours before serving.

Prep Time: 10 minutes
Cook Time: 20 minutes (churning)
Servings: 4

7. Banana Ice Cream

Ingredients:

- 3 ripe bananas, sliced

- 2 cups heavy cream

- 1 cup whole milk

- 1/2 cup sugar

- 1 tsp lemon juice

Directions:

- Blend bananas with lemon juice until smooth.

- In a bowl, mix heavy cream, milk, and sugar.

- Stir in the banana puree.

- Pour into an ice cream maker and churn as per instructions.

- Freeze for 2 hours before serving.

Prep Time: 15 minutes

Cook Time: 20 minutes (churning)
Servings: 4

8. Coffee Ice Cream

Ingredients:

- 2 cups heavy cream

- 1 cup whole milk

- 3/4 cup sugar

- 2 tbsp instant coffee granules

- 1 tsp vanilla extract

Directions:

- In a saucepan, heat milk and sugar until sugar dissolves.

- Stir in coffee granules until dissolved.

- Remove from heat and mix in heavy cream and vanilla extract.

- Chill the mixture in the refrigerator for 2 hours.

- Pour into an ice cream maker and churn as per instructions.

- Freeze for 2 hours before serving.

Prep Time: 15 minutes
Cook Time: 20 minutes (churning)
Servings: 4

9. Mango Ice Cream

Ingredients:

- 2 cups fresh mango, peeled and chopped

- 2 cups heavy cream

- 1 cup whole milk

- 3/4 cup sugar

- 1 tsp lemon juice

Directions:

- Blend mangoes with lemon juice and sugar until smooth.

- In a bowl, mix heavy cream and milk.

- Stir in the mango puree.

- Pour into an ice cream maker and churn as per instructions.

- Freeze for 2 hours before serving.

Prep Time: 15 minutes
Cook Time: 20 minutes (churning)
Servings: 4

10. Peanut Butter Ice Cream

Ingredients:

- 2 cups heavy cream

- 1 cup whole milk

- 3/4 cup sugar

- 1/2 cup peanut butter

- 1 tsp vanilla extract

Directions:

- In a bowl, mix heavy cream, milk, sugar, peanut butter, and vanilla extract until smooth.

- Pour into an ice cream maker and churn as per instructions.

- Freeze for 2 hours before serving.

Prep Time: 10 minutes
Cook Time: 20 minutes (churning)
Servings: 4

11. Lemon Ice Cream

Ingredients:

- 2 cups heavy cream

- 1 cup whole milk

- 3/4 cup sugar

- 1/4 cup lemon juice

- 1 tbsp lemon zest

Directions:

- In a bowl, mix heavy cream, milk, sugar, lemon juice, and lemon zest.

- Pour into an ice cream maker and churn as per instructions.

- Freeze for 2 hours before serving.

Prep Time: 10 minutes
Cook Time: 20 minutes (churning)
Servings: 4

12. Coconut Ice Cream

Ingredients:

- 2 cups coconut milk

- 1 cup heavy cream

- 3/4 cup sugar

- 1 tsp vanilla extract

Directions:

- In a bowl, mix coconut milk, heavy cream, sugar, and vanilla extract.

- Pour into an ice cream maker and churn as per instructions.

- Freeze for 2 hours before serving.

Prep Time: 10 minutes
Cook Time: 20 minutes (churning)
Servings: 4

13. Pistachio Ice Cream

Ingredients:

- 2 cups heavy cream

- 1 cup whole milk

- 3/4 cup sugar

- 1/2 cup shelled pistachios, chopped

- 1/2 tsp almond extract

Directions:

- In a bowl, mix heavy cream, milk, sugar, and almond extract.

- Pour into an ice cream maker and churn as per instructions.

- Add chopped pistachios in the last 5 minutes of churning.

- Freeze for 2 hours before serving.

Prep Time: 10 minutes
Cook Time: 20 minutes (churning)
Servings: 4

14. Blueberry Ice Cream

Ingredients:

- 2 cups fresh blueberries

- 2 cups heavy cream

- 1 cup whole milk

- 3/4 cup sugar

- 1 tsp lemon juice

Directions:

- Blend blueberries with lemon juice and sugar until smooth.

- In a bowl, mix heavy cream and milk.

- Stir in the blueberry puree.

- Pour into an ice cream maker and churn as per instructions.

- Freeze for 2 hours before serving.

Prep Time: 15 minutes
Cook Time: 20 minutes (churning)
Servings: 4

15. Honey Lavender Ice Cream

Ingredients:

- 2 cups heavy cream

- 1 cup whole milk

- 3/4 cup honey

- 1 tbsp dried lavender flowers

- 1 tsp vanilla extract

Directions:

- In a saucepan, heat milk, honey, and lavender flowers until the honey dissolves.

- Remove from heat and let steep for 15 minutes.

- Strain the mixture, then stir in heavy cream and vanilla extract.

- Chill in the refrigerator for 2 hours.

- Pour into an ice cream maker and churn as per instructions.

- Freeze for 2 hours before serving.

Prep Time: 20 minutes
Cook Time: 20 minutes (churning)
Servings: 4

16. Matcha Green Tea Ice Cream

Ingredients:

- 2 cups heavy cream

- 1 cup whole milk

- 3/4 cup sugar

- 2 tbsp matcha green tea powder

- 1 tsp vanilla extract

Directions:

- In a bowl, mix heavy cream, milk, sugar, matcha powder, and vanilla extract until smooth.

- Pour into an ice cream maker and churn as per instructions.

- Freeze for 2 hours before serving.

Prep Time: 10 minutes
Cook Time: 20 minutes (churning)
Servings: 4

17. Maple Walnut Ice Cream

Ingredients:

- 2 cups heavy cream

- 1 cup whole milk

- 3/4 cup maple syrup

- 1/2 cup chopped walnuts

- 1 tsp vanilla extract

Directions:

- In a bowl, mix heavy cream, milk, and maple syrup.

- Pour into an ice cream maker and churn as per instructions.

- Add chopped walnuts in the last 5 minutes of churning.

- Freeze for 2 hours before serving.

Prep Time: 10 minutes
Cook Time: 20 minutes (churning)
Servings: 4

18. Rocky Road Ice Cream

Ingredients:

- 2 cups heavy cream

- 1 cup whole milk

- 3/4 cup sugar

- 1/2 cup cocoa powder

- 1 cup mini marshmallows

- 1/2 cup chopped almonds

- 1 tsp vanilla extract

Directions:

- In a saucepan, heat milk, sugar, and cocoa powder until sugar dissolves.

- Remove from heat and mix in heavy cream and vanilla extract.

- Chill the mixture in the refrigerator for 2 hours.

- Pour into an ice cream maker and churn as per instructions.

- Add marshmallows and almonds in the last 5 minutes of churning.

- Freeze for 2 hours before serving.

Prep Time: 20 minutes
Cook Time: 20 minutes (churning)
Servings: 4

19. Caramel Apple Ice Cream

Ingredients:

- 2 cups heavy cream

- 1 cup whole milk

- 3/4 cup sugar

- 1/2 cup caramel sauce

- 1 cup apple pie filling, chopped

- 1 tsp cinnamon

Directions:

- In a bowl, mix heavy cream, milk, sugar, caramel sauce, and cinnamon.

- Pour into an ice cream maker and churn as per instructions.

- Add chopped apple pie filling in the last 5 minutes of churning.

- Freeze for 2 hours before serving.

Prep Time: 15 minutes
Cook Time: 20 minutes (churning)
Servings: 4

20. Black Sesame Ice Cream

Ingredients:

- 2 cups heavy cream

- 1 cup whole milk

- 3/4 cup sugar

- 1/2 cup black sesame seeds, toasted and ground

- 1 tsp vanilla extract

Directions:

- In a bowl, mix heavy cream, milk, sugar, ground black sesame seeds, and vanilla extract.

- Pour into an ice cream maker and churn as per instructions.

- Freeze for 2 hours before serving.

Prep Time: 15 minutes
Cook Time: 20 minutes (churning)
Servings: 4

Enjoy making and tasting these wonderful ice cream flavors!

Chapter 4

Creamiccino Recipes

Here are 20 delicious Creamiccino recipes for you:

1. Vanilla Bean Creamiccino

Ingredients:

- 1 cup strong brewed coffee, chilled

- 1 cup milk

- 1/4 cup heavy cream

- 1/4 cup sugar

- 1 tsp vanilla extract

- Ice cubes

Directions:

- Combine coffee, milk, heavy cream, sugar, and vanilla extract in a blender.

- Add a handful of ice cubes.

- Blend until smooth and frothy.

- Pour into glasses and serve immediately.

Prep Time: 5 minutes
Cook Time: 0 minutes
Servings: 2

2. Caramel Creamiccino

Ingredients:

- 1 cup strong brewed coffee, chilled

- 1 cup milk

- 1/4 cup caramel sauce

- 1/4 cup heavy cream

- Ice cubes

Directions:

- Mix coffee, milk, caramel sauce, and heavy cream in a blender.

- Add ice cubes and blend until smooth.

- Drizzle extra caramel sauce on top if desired.

- Serve immediately.

Prep Time: 5 minutes
Cook Time: 0 minutes
Servings: 2

3. Mocha Creamiccino

Ingredients:

- 1 cup strong brewed coffee, chilled

- 1 cup milk

* 1/4 cup heavy cream

* 2 tbsp cocoa powder

* 1/4 cup sugar

* Ice cubes

Directions:

* Combine coffee, milk, heavy cream, cocoa powder, and sugar in a blender.

* Add ice cubes and blend until creamy.

* Pour into glasses and serve.

Prep Time: 5 minutes
Cook Time: 0 minutes
Servings: 2

4. Hazelnut Creamiccino

Ingredients:

- 1 cup strong brewed coffee, chilled

- 1 cup milk

- 1/4 cup hazelnut syrup

- 1/4 cup heavy cream

- Ice cubes

Directions:

- Blend coffee, milk, hazelnut syrup, and heavy cream.

- Add ice cubes and blend until smooth.

- Serve in chilled glasses.

Prep Time: 5 minutes
Cook Time: 0 minutes
Servings: 2

5. Cinnamon Creamiccino

Ingredients:

- 1 cup strong brewed coffee, chilled

- 1 cup milk

- 1/4 cup heavy cream

- 1/4 cup sugar

- 1 tsp ground cinnamon

- Ice cubes

Directions:

- Mix coffee, milk, heavy cream, sugar, and ground cinnamon in a blender.

- Add ice cubes and blend until frothy.

- Pour into glasses and sprinkle extra cinnamon on top.

Prep Time: 5 minutes
Cook Time: 0 minutes
Servings: 2

6. Almond Creamiccino

Ingredients:

- 1 cup strong brewed coffee, chilled

- 1 cup almond milk

- 1/4 cup heavy cream

- 1/4 cup sugar

- 1 tsp almond extract

- Ice cubes

Directions:

- Combine coffee, almond milk, heavy cream, sugar, and almond extract in a blender.

- Add ice cubes and blend until smooth.

- Serve immediately.

Prep Time: 5 minutes
Cook Time: 0 minutes
Servings: 2

7. Coconut Creamiccino

Ingredients:

- 1 cup strong brewed coffee, chilled

- 1 cup coconut milk

- 1/4 cup heavy cream

- 1/4 cup sugar

- Ice cubes

Directions:

- Blend coffee, coconut milk, heavy cream, and sugar.

- Add ice cubes and blend until creamy.

- Serve in chilled glasses.

Prep Time: 5 minutes
Cook Time: 0 minutes
Servings: 2

8. Mint Creamiccino

Ingredients:

- 1 cup strong brewed coffee, chilled

- 1 cup milk

- 1/4 cup heavy cream

- 1/4 cup sugar

- 1 tsp peppermint extract

- Ice cubes

Directions:

- Combine coffee, milk, heavy cream, sugar, and peppermint extract in a blender.

- Add ice cubes and blend until frothy.

- Serve immediately.

Prep Time: 5 minutes
Cook Time: 0 minutes
Servings: 2

9. Pumpkin Spice Creamiccino

Ingredients:

- 1 cup strong brewed coffee, chilled

- 1 cup milk

- 1/4 cup heavy cream

- 1/4 cup sugar

- 1 tbsp pumpkin puree

- 1/2 tsp pumpkin spice

- Ice cubes

Directions:

- Mix coffee, milk, heavy cream, sugar, pumpkin puree, and pumpkin spice in a blender.

- Add ice cubes and blend until smooth.

- Serve immediately.

Prep Time: 5 minutes
Cook Time: 0 minutes
Servings: 2

10. White Chocolate Creamiccino

Ingredients:

- 1 cup strong brewed coffee, chilled

- 1 cup milk

- 1/4 cup heavy cream

- 1/4 cup white chocolate syrup

- Ice cubes

Directions:

- Blend coffee, milk, heavy cream, and white chocolate syrup.

- Add ice cubes and blend until creamy.

- Serve immediately.

Prep Time: 5 minutes
Cook Time: 0 minutes
Servings: 2

11. Peanut Butter Creamiccino

Ingredients:

- 1 cup strong brewed coffee, chilled

- 1 cup milk

- 1/4 cup heavy cream

- 2 tbsp peanut butter

- 1/4 cup sugar

- Ice cubes

Directions:

- Combine coffee, milk, heavy cream, peanut butter, and sugar in a blender.

- Add ice cubes and blend until smooth.

- Serve immediately.

Prep Time: 5 minutes
Cook Time: 0 minutes
Servings: 2

12. Maple Creamiccino

Ingredients:

- 1 cup strong brewed coffee, chilled

- 1 cup milk

- 1/4 cup heavy cream

- 1/4 cup maple syrup

- Ice cubes

Directions:

- Mix coffee, milk, heavy cream, and maple syrup in a blender.

- Add ice cubes and blend until frothy.

- Serve immediately.

Prep Time: 5 minutes
Cook Time: 0 minutes
Servings: 2

13. Honey Lavender Creamiccino

Ingredients:

- 1 cup strong brewed coffee, chilled

- 1 cup milk

- 1/4 cup heavy cream

- 2 tbsp honey

- 1/2 tsp lavender extract

- Ice cubes

Directions:

- Blend coffee, milk, heavy cream, honey, and lavender extract.

- Add ice cubes and blend until creamy.

- Serve immediately.

Prep Time: 5 minutes
Cook Time: 0 minutes
Servings: 2

14. Chai Spice Creamiccino

Ingredients:

- 1 cup strong brewed coffee, chilled

- 1 cup milk

- 1/4 cup heavy cream

- 1/4 cup sugar

- 1 tsp chai spice blend

- Ice cubes

Directions:

- Combine coffee, milk, heavy cream, sugar, and chai spice blend in a blender.

- Add ice cubes and blend until smooth.

- Serve immediately.

Prep Time: 5 minutes
Cook Time: 0 minutes
Servings: 2

15. Salted Caramel Creamiccino

Ingredients:

- 1 cup strong brewed coffee, chilled

- 1 cup milk

- 1/4 cup heavy cream

- 1/4 cup salted caramel sauce

- Ice cubes

Directions:

- Mix coffee, milk, heavy cream, and salted caramel sauce in a blender.

- Add ice cubes and blend until frothy.

- Serve immediately.

Prep Time: 5 minutes
Cook Time: 0 minutes
Servings: 2

16. Raspberry Creamiccino

Ingredients:

- 1 cup strong brewed coffee, chilled

- 1 cup milk

- 1/4 cup heavy cream

- 1/4 cup raspberry syrup

Directions:

- Blend coffee, milk, heavy cream, and raspberry syrup.

- Add ice cubes and blend until creamy.

- Serve immediately.

Prep Time: 5 minutes
Cook Time: 0 minutes
Servings: 2

17. Banana Creamiccino

Ingredients:

- 1 cup strong brewed coffee, chilled

- 1 cup milk

- 1/4 cup heavy cream

- 1 ripe banana

- 1/4 cup sugar

- Ice cubes

Directions:

- Combine coffee, milk, heavy cream, banana, and sugar in a blender.

- Add ice cubes and blend until smooth.

- Serve immediately.

Prep Time: 5 minutes
Cook Time: 0 minutes
Servings: 2
18. Oreo Creamiccino

Ingredients:

- 1 cup strong brewed coffee, chilled

- 1 cup milk

- 1/4 cup heavy cream

- 4 Oreo cookies

- 1/4 cup sugar

- Ice cubes

Directions:

- Blend coffee, milk, heavy cream, Oreo cookies, and sugar.

- Add ice cubes and blend until creamy.

- Serve immediately.

Prep Time: 5 minutes
Cook Time: 0 minutes
Servings: 2

19. Mocha Coconut Creamiccino

Ingredients:

- 1 cup strong brewed coffee, chilled

- 1 cup coconut milk

- 1/4 cup heavy cream

- 2 tbsp cocoa powder

- 1/4 cup sugar

- Ice cubes

Directions:

- Combine coffee, coconut milk, heavy cream, cocoa powder, and sugar in a blender.

- Add ice cubes and blend until smooth.

- Serve immediately.

Prep Time: 5 minutes
Cook Time: 0 minutes

Servings: 2

20. Matcha Creamiccino

Ingredients:

- 1 cup strong brewed coffee, chilled

- 1 cup milk

- 1/4 cup heavy cream

- 2 tsp matcha powder

- 1/4 cup sugar

- Ice cubes

Directions:

- Blend coffee, milk, heavy cream, matcha powder, and sugar.

- Add ice cubes and blend until creamy.

- Serve immediately.

Prep Time: 5 minutes
Cook Time: 0 minutes
Servings: 2

Enjoy these delicious Creamiccino recipes!

Chapter 5

Sorbet Recipes

Here are 20 refreshing sorbet recipes for you to enjoy:

1. Lemon Sorbet

Ingredients:

- 2 cups water

- 1 cup sugar

- 1 cup fresh lemon juice (about 4-5 lemons)

- 1 tbsp lemon zest

Directions:

- In a saucepan, heat water and sugar until sugar dissolves.

- Remove from heat and let it cool.

- Add lemon juice and zest to the mixture.

- Pour into a container and freeze for 4-6 hours, stirring every hour to break up ice crystals.

Prep Time: 10 minutes

Cook Time: 0 minutes

Servings: 4

2. Strawberry Sorbet

Ingredients:

- 4 cups fresh strawberries, hulled

- 1 cup sugar

- 1 cup water

- 1 tbsp lemon juice

Directions:

- Blend strawberries until smooth.

- In a saucepan, heat water and sugar until sugar dissolves.

- Mix the strawberry puree, lemon juice, and sugar water.

- Pour into a container and freeze for 4-6 hours, stirring every hour.

Prep Time: 15 minutes
Cook Time: 0 minutes
Servings: 4

3. Mango Sorbet

Ingredients:

- 4 cups fresh mango, peeled and chopped

- 1 cup sugar

- 1 cup water

- 1 tbsp lime juice

Directions:

- Blend mango until smooth.

- In a saucepan, heat water and sugar until sugar dissolves.

- Mix the mango puree, lime juice, and sugar water.

- Pour into a container and freeze for 4-6 hours, stirring every hour.

Prep Time: 15 minutes
Cook Time: 0 minutes
Servings: 4

4. Raspberry Sorbet

Ingredients:

- 4 cups fresh raspberries

- 1 cup sugar

- 1 cup water

- 1 tbsp lemon juice

Directions:

- Blend raspberries until smooth and strain to remove seeds.

- In a saucepan, heat water and sugar until sugar dissolves.

- Mix the raspberry puree, lemon juice, and sugar water.

- Pour into a container and freeze for 4-6 hours, stirring every hour.

Prep Time: 20 minutes
Cook Time: 0 minutes
Servings: 4

5. Pineapple Sorbet

Ingredients:

- 4 cups fresh pineapple, chopped

- 1 cup sugar

- 1 cup water

- 1 tbsp lime juice

Directions:

- Blend pineapple until smooth.

- In a saucepan, heat water and sugar until sugar dissolves.

- Mix the pineapple puree, lime juice, and sugar water.

- Pour into a container and freeze for 4-6 hours, stirring every hour.

Prep Time: 15 minutes
Cook Time: 0 minutes
Servings: 4

6. Watermelon Sorbet

Ingredients:

- 4 cups watermelon, seeded and chopped

- 1 cup sugar

- 1 cup water

- 1 tbsp lime juice

Directions:

- Blend watermelon until smooth.

- In a saucepan, heat water and sugar until sugar dissolves.

- Mix the watermelon puree, lime juice, and sugar water.

- Pour into a container and freeze for 4-6 hours, stirring every hour.

Prep Time: 15 minutes
Cook Time: 0 minutes
Servings: 4

7. Blueberry Sorbet

Ingredients:

- 4 cups fresh blueberries

- 1 cup sugar

- 1 cup water

- 1 tbsp lemon juice

Directions:

- Blend blueberries until smooth.

- In a saucepan, heat water and sugar until sugar dissolves.

- Mix the blueberry puree, lemon juice, and sugar water.

- Pour into a container and freeze for 4-6 hours, stirring every hour.

Prep Time: 15 minutes
Cook Time: 0 minutes
Servings: 4

8. Peach Sorbet

Ingredients:

- 4 cups fresh peaches, peeled and chopped

- 1 cup sugar

- 1 cup water

- 1 tbsp lemon juice

Directions:

- Blend peaches until smooth.

- In a saucepan, heat water and sugar until sugar dissolves.

- Mix the peach puree, lemon juice, and sugar water.

- Pour into a container and freeze for 4-6 hours, stirring every hour.

Prep Time: 15 minutes
Cook Time: 0 minutes
Servings: 4

9. Orange Sorbet

Ingredients:

- 2 cups fresh orange juice (about 4-5 oranges)

- 1 cup water

- 1 cup sugar

- 1 tbsp orange zest

Directions:

- In a saucepan, heat water and sugar until sugar dissolves.

- Remove from heat and let it cool.

- Add orange juice and zest to the mixture.

- Pour into a container and freeze for 4-6 hours, stirring every hour to break up ice crystals.

Prep Time: 10 minutes
Cook Time: 0 minutes
Servings: 4

10. Kiwi Sorbet

Ingredients:

- 6 kiwis, peeled and chopped

- 1 cup sugar

- 1 cup water

- 1 tbsp lemon juice

Directions:

- Blend kiwis until smooth.

- In a saucepan, heat water and sugar until sugar dissolves.

- Mix the kiwi puree, lemon juice, and sugar water.

- Pour into a container and freeze for 4-6 hours, stirring every hour.

Prep Time: 15 minutes
Cook Time: 0 minutes
Servings: 4

11. Apple Sorbet

Ingredients:

- 4 cups apple juice

- 1 cup sugar

- 1 tbsp lemon juice

Directions:

- In a saucepan, heat apple juice and sugar until sugar dissolves.

- Remove from heat and let it cool.

- Add lemon juice.

- Pour into a container and freeze for 4-6 hours, stirring every hour to break up ice crystals.

Prep Time: 10 minutes

Servings: 4

12. Lime Sorbet

Ingredients:

- 2 cups water

- 1 cup sugar

- 1 cup fresh lime juice (about 8-10 limes)

- 1 tbsp lime zest

Directions:

- In a saucepan, heat water and sugar until sugar dissolves.

- Remove from heat and let it cool.

- Add lime juice and zest to the mixture.

- Pour into a container and freeze for 4-6 hours, stirring every hour to break up ice crystals.

Prep Time: 10 minutes
Cook Time: 0 minutes
Servings: 4

13. Grape Sorbet

Ingredients:

- 4 cups seedless grapes

- 1 cup sugar

- 1 cup water

- 1 tbsp lemon juice

Directions:

- Blend grapes until smooth and strain to remove skins.

- In a saucepan, heat water and sugar until sugar dissolves.

- Mix the grape puree, lemon juice, and sugar water.

- Pour into a container and freeze for 4-6 hours, stirring every hour.

Prep Time: 20 minutes
Cook Time: 0 minutes
Servings: 4

14. Cantaloupe Sorbet

Ingredients:

- 4 cups cantaloupe, chopped

- 1 cup sugar

- 1 cup water

- 1 tbsp lemon juice

Directions:

- Blend cantaloupe until smooth.

- In a saucepan, heat water and sugar until sugar dissolves.

- Mix the cantaloupe puree, lemon juice, and sugar water.

- Pour into a container and freeze for 4-6 hours, stirring every hour.

Prep Time: 15 minutes
Cook Time: 0 minutes
Servings: 4

15. Blackberry Sorbet

Ingredients:

- 4 cups fresh blackberries

- 1 cup sugar

- 1 cup water

- 1 tbsp lemon juice

Directions:

- Blend blackberries until smooth and strain to remove seeds.

- In a saucepan, heat water and sugar until sugar dissolves.

- Mix the blackberry puree, lemon juice, and sugar water.

- Pour into a container and freeze for 4-6 hours, stirring every hour.

Prep Time: 20 minutes
Cook Time: 0 minutes
Servings: 4

16. Cranberry Sorbet

Ingredients:

- 4 cups fresh cranberries

- 1 cup sugar

- 1 cup water

- 1 tbsp orange juice

Directions:

- Blend cranberries until smooth.

- In a saucepan, heat water and sugar until sugar dissolves.

- Mix the cranberry puree and orange juice with sugar water.

- Pour into a container and freeze for 4-6 hours, stirring every hour.

Prep Time: 20 minutes
Cook Time: 0 minutes
Servings: 4

17. Papaya Sorbet

Ingredients:

- 4 cups fresh papaya, peeled and chopped

- 1 cup of sugar

- 1 cup of water

- 1 tbsp lime juice

Directions:

- Blend papaya until smooth.

- In a saucepan, heat water and sugar until sugar dissolves.

- Mix the papaya puree, lime juice, and sugar water.

- Pour into a container and freeze for 4-6 hours, stirring every hour.

Prep Time: 15 minutes
Cook Time: 0 minutes
Servings: 4

18. Pomegranate Sorbet

Ingredients:

- 4 cups fresh pomegranate juice

- 1 cup of sugar

- 1 tbsp lemon juice

Directions:

- In a saucepan, heat pomegranate juice and sugar until sugar dissolves.

- Remove from heat and let it cool.

- Add lemon juice.

- Pour into a container and freeze for 4-6 hours, stirring every hour to break up ice crystals.

Prep Time: 10 minutes
Cook Time: 0 minutes

Servings: 4

19. Passion Fruit Sorbet

Ingredients:

- 4 cups passion fruit pulp

- 1 cup of sugar

- 1 cup of water

- 1 tbsp lemon juice

Directions:

- Blend passion fruit pulp until smooth.

- In a saucepan, heat water and sugar until sugar dissolves.

- Mix the passion fruit puree, lemon juice, and sugar water.

- Pour into a container and freeze for 4-6 hours, stirring every hour.

Prep Time: 15 minutes
Cook Time: 0 minutes
Servings: 4

20. Cherry Sorbet

Ingredients:

- 4 cups fresh cherries, pitted

- 1 cup of sugar

- 1 cup of water

- 1 tbsp lemon juice

Directions:

- Blend cherries until smooth and strain to remove skins.

- In a saucepan, heat water and sugar until sugar dissolves.

- Mix the cherry puree, lemon juice, and sugar water.

- Pour into a container and freeze for 4-6 hours, stirring every hour.

Prep Time: 20 minutes
Cook Time: 0 minutes
Servings: 4

Enjoy making and savoring these delicious sorbet recipes!

Chapter 6

Gelato Recipes

Here are 20 delicious gelato recipes for you:

1. Classic Vanilla Gelato

Ingredients:

- 2 cups whole milk

- 1 cup heavy cream

- 3/4 cup sugar

- 1 vanilla bean, split and scraped (or 1 tbsp vanilla extract)

- 5 egg yolks

Directions:

- In a saucepan, heat milk, cream, and vanilla bean (or extract) until just simmering.

- In a bowl, whisk sugar and egg yolks until pale.

- Gradually add hot milk mixture to egg yolks, whisking constantly.

- Return mixture to saucepan and cook over low heat until thickened.

- Strain the mixture and cool completely.

- Churn in an ice cream maker according to the manufacturer's instructions.

- Freeze for 2 hours before serving.

Prep Time: 15 minutes

Cook Time: 20 minutes

Servings: 4

2. Chocolate Gelato

Ingredients:

- 2 cups whole milk

- 1 cup heavy cream

- 3/4 cup sugar

- 1/2 cup cocoa powder

- 5 egg yolks

Directions:

- In a saucepan, heat milk, cream, and cocoa powder until just simmering.

- In a bowl, whisk sugar and egg yolks until pale.

- Gradually add hot milk mixture to egg yolks, whisking constantly.

- Return mixture to saucepan and cook over low heat until thickened.

- Strain the mixture and cool completely.

- Churn in an ice cream maker according to the manufacturer's instructions.

- Freeze for 2 hours before serving.

Prep Time: 15 minutes
Cook Time: 20 minutes
Servings: 4

3. Strawberry Gelato

Ingredients:

- 2 cups fresh strawberries, hulled and sliced

- 2 cups whole milk

- 1 cup heavy cream

- 3/4 cup sugar

- 5 egg yolks

Directions:

- Blend strawberries until smooth and strain to remove seeds.

- In a saucepan, heat milk and cream until just simmering.

- In a bowl, whisk sugar and egg yolks until pale.

- Gradually add hot milk mixture to egg yolks, whisking constantly.

- Return mixture to saucepan and cook over low heat until thickened.

- Mix in strawberry puree and cool completely.

- Churn in an ice cream maker according to the manufacturer's instructions.

- Freeze for 2 hours before serving.

Prep Time: 20 minutes
Cook Time: 20 minutes
Servings: 4

4. Pistachio Gelato

Ingredients:

- 2 cups whole milk

- 1 cup heavy cream

- 3/4 cup sugar

- 1 cup shelled pistachios, finely ground

- 5 egg yolks

Directions:

- In a saucepan, heat milk, cream, and ground pistachios until just simmering.

- In a bowl, whisk sugar and egg yolks until pale.

- Gradually add hot milk mixture to egg yolks, whisking constantly.

- Return mixture to saucepan and cook over low heat until thickened.

- Strain the mixture and cool completely.

- Churn in an ice cream maker according to the manufacturer's instructions.

- Freeze for 2 hours before serving.

Prep Time: 20 minutes
Cook Time: 20 minutes
Servings: 4

5. Hazelnut Gelato

Ingredients:

- 2 cups whole milk

- 1 cup heavy cream

- 3/4 cup sugar

- 1 cup hazelnuts, toasted and finely ground

- 5 egg yolks

Directions:

- In a saucepan, heat milk, cream, and ground hazelnuts until just simmering.

- In a bowl, whisk sugar and egg yolks until pale.

- Gradually add hot milk mixture to egg yolks, whisking constantly.

- Return mixture to saucepan and cook over low heat until thickened.

- Strain the mixture and cool completely.

- Churn in an ice cream maker according to the manufacturer's instructions.

- Freeze for 2 hours before serving.

Prep Time: 20 minutes
Cook Time: 20 minutes
Servings: 4

6. Coffee Gelato

Ingredients:

- 2 cups whole milk

- 1 cup heavy cream

- 3/4 cup sugar

- 1/4 cup instant coffee granules

- 5 egg yolks

Directions:

- In a saucepan, heat milk, cream, and coffee granules until just simmering.

- In a bowl, whisk sugar and egg yolks until pale.

- Gradually add hot milk mixture to egg yolks, whisking constantly.

- Return mixture to saucepan and cook over low heat until thickened.

- Strain the mixture and cool completely.

- Churn in an ice cream maker according to the manufacturer's instructions.

- Freeze for 2 hours before serving.

Prep Time: 15 minutes
Cook Time: 20 minutes
Servings: 4

7. Lemon Gelato

Ingredients:

- 2 cups whole milk

- 1 cup heavy cream

- 3/4 cup sugar

- 1/4 cup fresh lemon juice

- 1 tbsp lemon zest

- 5 egg yolks

Directions:

- In a saucepan, heat milk, cream, and lemon zest until just simmering.

- In a bowl, whisk sugar and egg yolks until pale.

- Gradually add hot milk mixture to egg yolks, whisking constantly.

- Return mixture to saucepan and cook over low heat until thickened.

- Strain the mixture and cool completely. Stir in lemon juice.

- Churn in an ice cream maker according to the manufacturer's instructions.

- Freeze for 2 hours before serving.

Prep Time: 15 minutes
Cook Time: 20 minutes
Servings: 4

8. Mango Gelato

Ingredients:

- 2 cups fresh mango, peeled and chopped

- 2 cups whole milk

- 1 cup heavy cream

- 3/4 cup sugar

- 5 egg yolks

Directions:

- Blend mango until smooth.

- In a saucepan, heat milk and cream until just simmering.

- In a bowl, whisk sugar and egg yolks until pale.

- Gradually add hot milk mixture to egg yolks, whisking constantly.

- Return mixture to saucepan and cook over low heat until thickened.

- Mix in mango puree and cool completely.

- Churn in an ice cream maker according to the manufacturer's instructions.

- Freeze for 2 hours before serving.

Prep Time: 20 minutes
Cook Time: 20 minutes
Servings: 4

9. Mint Chocolate Chip Gelato

Ingredients:

- 2 cups whole milk

- 1 cup heavy cream

- 3/4 cup sugar

- 1 tsp peppermint extract

- 1 cup chocolate chips

- 5 egg yolks

Directions:

- In a saucepan, heat milk, cream, and peppermint extract until just simmering.

- In a bowl, whisk sugar and egg yolks until pale.

- Gradually add hot milk mixture to egg yolks, whisking constantly.

- Return mixture to saucepan and cook over low heat until thickened.

- Strain the mixture and cool completely.

- Churn in an ice cream maker according to the manufacturer's instructions.

- Add chocolate chips during the last 5 minutes of churning.

- Freeze for 2 hours before serving.

Prep Time: 15 minutes
Cook Time: 20 minutes
Servings: 4

10. Coconut Gelato

Ingredients:

- 2 cups coconut milk

- 1 cup heavy cream

- 3/4 cup sugar

- 1 tsp vanilla extract

- 5 egg yolks

Directions:

- In a saucepan, heat coconut milk, cream, and vanilla extract until just simmering.

- In a bowl, whisk sugar and egg yolks until pale.

- Gradually add hot milk mixture to egg yolks, whisking constantly.

- Return mixture to saucepan and cook over low heat until thickened.

- Strain the mixture and cool completely.

- Churn in an ice cream maker according to the manufacturer's instructions.

- Freeze for 2 hours before serving.

Prep Time: 15 minutes
Cook Time: 20 minutes
Servings: 4

11. Caramel Gelato

Ingredients:

- 2 cups whole milk

- 1 cup heavy cream

- 1 cup sugar

- 5 egg yolks

- 1/2 cup caramel sauce

Directions:

- In a saucepan, heat milk and cream until just simmering.

- In another saucepan, melt sugar until it turns golden brown.

- Slowly add the hot milk mixture to the caramel, stirring constantly.

- In a bowl, whisk egg yolks until pale.

- Gradually add caramel mixture to egg yolks, whisking constantly.

- Return mixture to saucepan and cook over low heat until thickened.

- Strain the mixture and cool completely. Stir in caramel sauce.

- Churn in an ice cream maker according to the manufacturer's instructions.

- Freeze for 2 hours before serving.

Prep Time: 20 minutes
Cook Time: 20 minutes
Servings: 4

12. Tiramisu Gelato

Ingredients:

- 2 cups whole milk

- 1 cup heavy cream

- 3/4 cup sugar

- 1/4 cup instant coffee granules

- 1/4 cup marsala wine

- 5 egg yolks

- 1/2 cup mascarpone cheese

Directions:

- In a saucepan, heat milk, cream, and coffee granules until just simmering.

- In a bowl, whisk sugar and egg yolks until pale.

- Gradually add hot milk mixture to egg yolks, whisking constantly.

- Return mixture to saucepan and cook over low heat until thickened.

- Strain the mixture and cool completely. Stir in marsala wine and mascarpone cheese.

- Churn in an ice cream maker according to the manufacturer's instructions.

- Freeze for 2 hours before serving.

Prep Time: 20 minutes
Cook Time: 20 minutes
Servings: 4

13. Almond Gelato

Ingredients:

- 2 cups whole milk

- 1 cup heavy cream

- 3/4 cup sugar

- 1 cup almonds, toasted and finely ground

- 1 tsp almond extract

- 5 egg yolks

Directions:

- In a saucepan, heat milk, cream, and ground almonds until just simmering.

- In a bowl, whisk sugar and egg yolks until pale.

- Gradually add hot milk mixture to egg yolks, whisking constantly.

- Return mixture to saucepan and cook over low heat until thickened.

- Strain the mixture and cool completely. Stir in almond extract.

- Churn in an ice cream maker according to the manufacturer's instructions.

- Freeze for 2 hours before serving.

Prep Time: 20 minutes
Cook Time: 20 minutes
Servings: 4

14. Blackberry Gelato

Ingredients:

- 2 cups fresh blackberries

- 2 cups whole milk

- 1 cup heavy cream

- 3/4 cup sugar

- 5 egg yolks

Directions:

- Blend blackberries until smooth and strain to remove seeds.

- In a saucepan, heat milk and cream until just simmering.

- In a bowl, whisk sugar and egg yolks until pale.

- Gradually add hot milk mixture to egg yolks, whisking constantly.

- Return mixture to saucepan and cook over low heat until thickened.

- Mix in blackberry puree and cool completely.

- Churn in an ice cream maker according to the manufacturer's instructions.

- Freeze for 2 hours before serving.

Prep Time: 20 minutes

Cook Time: 20 minutes

Servings: 4

15. Matcha Green Tea Gelato

Ingredients:

- 2 cups whole milk

- 1 cup heavy cream

- 3/4 cup sugar

- 2 tbsp matcha green tea powder

- 5 egg yolks

Directions:

- In a saucepan, heat milk, cream, and matcha powder until just simmering.

- In a bowl, whisk sugar and egg yolks until pale.

- Gradually add hot milk mixture to egg yolks, whisking constantly.

- Return mixture to saucepan and cook over low heat until thickened.

- Strain the mixture and cool completely.

- Churn in an ice cream maker according to the manufacturer's instructions.

- Freeze for 2 hours before serving.

Prep Time: 15 minutes
Cook Time: 20 minutes
Servings: 4

16. Blueberry Gelato

Ingredients:

- 2 cups fresh blueberries

- 2 cups whole milk

- 1 cup heavy cream

- 3/4 cup sugar

- 5 egg yolks

Directions:

- Blend blueberries until smooth and strain to remove skins.

- In a saucepan, heat milk and cream until just simmering.

- In a bowl, whisk sugar and egg yolks until pale.

- Gradually add hot milk mixture to egg yolks, whisking constantly.

- Return mixture to saucepan and cook over low heat until thickened.

- Mix in blueberry puree and cool completely.

- Churn in an ice cream maker according to the manufacturer's instructions.

- Freeze for 2 hours before serving.

Prep Time: 20 minutes
Cook Time: 20 minutes
Servings: 4

17. Banana Gelato

Ingredients:

- 2 ripe bananas, mashed

- 2 cups whole milk

- 1 cup heavy cream

- 3/4 cup sugar

- 5 egg yolks

Directions:

- In a saucepan, heat milk and cream until just simmering.

- In a bowl, whisk sugar and egg yolks until pale.

- Gradually add hot milk mixture to egg yolks, whisking constantly.

- Return mixture to saucepan and cook over low heat until thickened.

- Mix in mashed bananas and cool completely.

- Churn in an ice cream maker according to the manufacturer's instructions.

- Freeze for 2 hours before serving.

Prep Time: 15 minutes
Cook Time: 20 minutes
Servings: 4

18. Raspberry Gelato

Ingredients:

- 2 cups fresh raspberries

- 2 cups whole milk

- 1 cup heavy cream

- 3/4 cup sugar

- 5 egg yolks

Directions:

- Blend raspberries until smooth and strain to remove seeds.

- In a saucepan, heat milk and cream until just simmering.

- In a bowl, whisk sugar and egg yolks until pale.

- Gradually add hot milk mixture to egg yolks, whisking constantly.

- Return mixture to saucepan and cook over low heat until thickened.

- Mix in raspberry puree and cool completely.

- Churn in an ice cream maker according to the manufacturer's instructions.

- Freeze for 2 hours before serving.

Prep Time: 20 minutes
Cook Time: 20 minutes
Servings: 4

19. Cinnamon Gelato

Ingredients:

- 2 cups whole milk

- 1 cup heavy cream

- 3/4 cup sugar

- 2 tsp ground cinnamon

- 5 egg yolks

Directions:

- In a saucepan, heat milk, cream, and ground cinnamon until just simmering.

- In a bowl, whisk sugar and egg yolks until pale.

- Gradually add hot milk mixture to egg yolks, whisking constantly.

- Return mixture to saucepan and cook over low heat until thickened.

- Strain the mixture and cool completely.

- Churn in an ice cream maker according to the manufacturer's instructions.

- Freeze for 2 hours before serving.

Prep Time: 15 minutes
Cook Time: 20 minutes
Servings: 4

20. Honey Gelato

Ingredients:

- 2 cups whole milk

- 1 cup heavy cream

- 3/4 cup honey

- 5 egg yolks

Directions:

- In a saucepan, heat milk, cream, and honey until just simmering.

- In a bowl, whisk egg yolks until pale.

- Gradually add hot milk mixture to egg yolks, whisking constantly.

- Return mixture to saucepan and cook over low heat until thickened.

- Strain the mixture and cool completely.

- Churn in an ice cream maker according to the manufacturer's instructions.

- Freeze for 2 hours before serving.

Prep Time: 15 minutes
Cook Time: 20 minutes
Servings: 4

Enjoy making and savoring these delightful gelato recipes!

Chapter 7

Smoothie Recipes

Here are 20 delicious smoothie recipes for you:

1. Strawberry Banana Smoothie

Ingredients:

- 1 cup fresh strawberries, hulled

- 1 ripe banana

- 1 cup plain yogurt

- 1/2 cup milk

- 1 tbsp honey (optional)

Directions:

- Place all ingredients in a blender.

- Blend until smooth.

- Pour into a glass and enjoy!

Prep Time: 5 minutes
Cook Time: 0 minutes
Servings: 1

2. Blueberry Spinach Smoothie

Ingredients:

- 1 cup fresh blueberries

- 1 cup fresh spinach

- 1 banana

- 1 cup almond milk

- 1 tbsp chia seeds (optional)

Directions:

- Place all ingredients in a blender.

- Blend until smooth.

- Pour into a glass and enjoy!

Prep Time: 5 minutes
Cook Time: 0 minutes
Servings: 1

3. Tropical Mango Smoothie

Ingredients:

- 1 cup fresh mango, peeled and chopped

- 1/2 cup pineapple chunks

- 1/2 cup coconut milk

- 1/2 cup orange juice

Directions:

- Place all ingredients in a blender.

- Blend until smooth.

- Pour into a glass and enjoy!

Prep Time: 5 minutes
Cook Time: 0 minutes
Servings: 1

4. Peanut Butter Banana Smoothie

Ingredients:

- 1 ripe banana

- 2 tbsp peanut butter

- 1 cup milk

- 1 tbsp honey (optional)

- 1/2 cup ice

Directions:

- Place all ingredients in a blender.

- Blend until smooth.

- Pour into a glass and enjoy!

Prep Time: 5 minutes
Cook Time: 0 minutes
Servings: 1

5. Green Detox Smoothie

Ingredients:

- 1 cup fresh spinach

- 1/2 cucumber, chopped

- 1 green apple, chopped

- 1/2 lemon, juiced

- 1 cup water

Directions:

- Place all ingredients in a blender.

- Blend until smooth.

- Pour into a glass and enjoy!

Prep Time: 5 minutes
Cook Time: 0 minutes
Servings: 1

6. Chocolate Avocado Smoothie

Ingredients:

- 1 ripe avocado

- 1 banana

- 2 tbsp cocoa powder

- 1 cup almond milk

- 1 tbsp honey (optional)

Directions:

- Place all ingredients in a blender.

- Blend until smooth.

- Pour into a glass and enjoy!

Prep Time: 5 minutes
Cook Time: 0 minutes
Servings: 1

7. Berry Blast Smoothie

Ingredients:

- 1/2 cup strawberries

- 1/2 cup blueberries

- 1/2 cup raspberries

- 1 cup plain yogurt

- 1/2 cup orange juice

Directions:

- Place all ingredients in a blender.

- Blend until smooth.

- Pour into a glass and enjoy!

Prep Time: 5 minutes

Cook Time: 0 minutes

Servings: 1

8. Pineapple Coconut Smoothie

Ingredients:

- 1 cup pineapple chunks

- 1/2 cup coconut milk

- 1/2 cup plain yogurt

- 1 tbsp honey (optional)

- 1/2 cup ice

Directions:

- Place all ingredients in a blender.

- Blend until smooth.

- Pour into a glass and enjoy!

Prep Time: 5 minutes
Cook Time: 0 minutes
Servings: 1

9. Orange Carrot Smoothie

Ingredients:

- 2 medium carrots, peeled and chopped

- 1 orange, peeled and segmented

- 1/2 cup orange juice

- 1/2 cup water

- 1 tbsp honey (optional)

Directions:

- Place all ingredients in a blender.

- Blend until smooth.

- Pour into a glass and enjoy!

Prep Time: 5 minutes
Servings: 1
10. Apple Cinnamon Smoothie

Ingredients:

- 1 apple, chopped

- 1 banana

- 1/2 tsp ground cinnamon

- 1 cup milk

- 1/2 cup plain yogurt

Directions:

- Place all ingredients in a blender.

- Blend until smooth.

- Pour into a glass and enjoy!

Prep Time: 5 minutes
Cook Time: 0 minutes
Servings: 1

11. Kiwi Spinach Smoothie

Ingredients:

- 2 kiwis, peeled and chopped

- 1 cup fresh spinach

- 1 banana

- 1 cup orange juice

- 1 tbsp chia seeds (optional)

Directions:

- Place all ingredients in a blender.

- Blend until smooth.

- Pour into a glass and enjoy!

Prep Time: 5 minutes
Cook Time: 0 minutes
Servings: 1

12. Mixed Berry Oat Smoothie

Ingredients:

- 1/2 cup mixed berries (strawberries, blueberries, raspberries)

- 1/2 cup oats

- 1 banana

- 1 cup almond milk

- 1 tbsp honey (optional)

Directions:

- Place all ingredients in a blender.

- Blend until smooth.

- Pour into a glass and enjoy!

Prep Time: 5 minutes
Cook Time: 0 minutes
Servings: 1

13. Peach Mango Smoothie

Ingredients:

- 1 cup fresh peaches, sliced

- 1 cup fresh mango, chopped

- 1 cup plain yogurt

- 1/2 cup orange juice

Directions:

- Place all ingredients in a blender.

- Blend until smooth.

- Pour into a glass and enjoy!

Prep Time: 5 minutes
Cook Time: 0 minutes
Servings: 1

14. Chocolate Banana Smoothie

Ingredients:

- 1 ripe banana

- 2 tbsp cocoa powder

- 1 cup milk

- 1 tbsp honey (optional)

- 1/2 cup ice

Directions:

- Place all ingredients in a blender.

- Blend until smooth.

- Pour into a glass and enjoy!

Prep Time: 5 minutes
Cook Time: 0 minutes
Servings: 1

15. Avocado Spinach Smoothie

Ingredients:

- 1 ripe avocado

- 1 cup fresh spinach

- 1 banana

- 1 cup almond milk

- 1 tbsp honey (optional)

Directions:

- Place all ingredients in a blender.

- Blend until smooth.

- Pour into a glass and enjoy!

Prep Time: 5 minutes
Cook Time: 0 minutes
Servings: 1

16. Coconut Blueberry Smoothie

Ingredients:

- 1 cup fresh blueberries

- 1/2 cup coconut milk

- 1/2 cup plain yogurt

- 1 tbsp honey (optional)

- 1/2 cup ice

Directions:

- Place all ingredients in a blender.

- Blend until smooth.

- Pour into a glass and enjoy!

Prep Time: 5 minutes
Cook Time: 0 minutes
Servings: 1

17. Watermelon Mint Smoothie

Ingredients:

- 2 cups watermelon, cubed and seeded

- 1/4 cup fresh mint leaves

- 1/2 cup water

- 1 tbsp lime juice

- 1 tbsp honey (optional)

Directions:

- Place all ingredients in a blender.

- Blend until smooth.

- Pour into a glass and enjoy!

Prep Time: 5 minutes
Cook Time: 0 minutes
Servings: 1

18. Pineapple Kale Smoothie

Ingredients:

- 1 cup pineapple chunks
- 1 cup fresh kale
- 1 banana
- 1 cup coconut water
- 1 tbsp chia seeds (optional)

Directions:

- Place all ingredients in a blender.
- Blend until smooth.
- Pour into a glass and enjoy!

Prep Time: 5 minutes
Cook Time: 0 minutes
Servings: 1

19. Raspberry Lemon Smoothie

Ingredients:

- 1 cup fresh raspberries

- 1 banana

- 1/2 cup plain yogurt

- 1/2 cup lemon juice

- 1 tbsp honey (optional)

Directions:

- Place all ingredients in a blender.

- Blend until smooth.

- Pour into a glass and enjoy!

Prep Time: 5 minutes
Cook Time: 0 minutes

Servings: 1

20. Chocolate Mint Smoothie

Ingredients:

- 1 ripe banana

- 2 tbsp cocoa powder

- 1/4 cup fresh mint leaves

- 1 cup milk

- 1 tbsp honey (optional)

Directions:

- Place all ingredients in a blender.

- Blend until smooth.

- Pour into a glass and enjoy!

Prep Time: 5 minutes
Cook Time: 0 minutes
Servings: 1

Enjoy making and savoring these delicious and nutritious smoothies!

Chapter 8

Milkshakes Recipes

Here are 20 delicious milkshake recipes:

1. Classic Vanilla Milkshake

Ingredients:

- 2 cups vanilla ice cream

- 1 cup milk

- 1 tsp vanilla extract

Directions:

- Place all ingredients in a blender.

- Blend until smooth.

- Pour into a glass and enjoy!

Prep Time: 5 minutes
Cook Time: 0 minutes
Servings: 1

2. Chocolate Milkshake

Ingredients:

- 2 cups chocolate ice cream

- 1 cup milk

- 2 tbsp chocolate syrup

Directions:

- Place all ingredients in a blender.

- Blend until smooth.

- Pour into a glass and enjoy!

Prep Time: 5 minutes
Cook Time: 0 minutes
Servings: 1

3. Strawberry Milkshake

Ingredients:

- 2 cups strawberry ice cream

- 1 cup milk

- 1/2 cup fresh strawberries

Directions:

- Place all ingredients in a blender.

- Blend until smooth.

- Pour into a glass and enjoy!

Prep Time: 5 minutes
Cook Time: 0 minutes
Servings: 1

4. Banana Milkshake

Ingredients:

- 2 cups vanilla ice cream

- 1 cup milk

- 1 ripe banana

Directions:

- Place all ingredients in a blender.

- Blend until smooth.

- Pour into a glass and enjoy!

Prep Time: 5 minutes
Cook Time: 0 minutes
Servings: 1

5. Peanut Butter Milkshake

Ingredients:

- 2 cups vanilla ice cream

- 1 cup milk

- 2 tbsp peanut butter

Directions:

- Place all ingredients in a blender.

- Blend until smooth.

- Pour into a glass and enjoy!

Prep Time: 5 minutes
Cook Time: 0 minutes
Servings: 1

6. Cookies and Cream Milkshake

Ingredients:

- 2 cups cookies and cream ice cream

- 1 cup milk

- 4 Oreo cookies

Directions:

- Place all ingredients in a blender.

- Blend until smooth.

- Pour into a glass and enjoy!

Prep Time: 5 minutes
Cook Time: 0 minutes
Servings: 1

7. Mint Chocolate Chip Milkshake

Ingredients:

- 2 cups mint chocolate chip ice cream

- 1 cup milk

- 1/2 tsp mint extract (optional)

Directions:

- Place all ingredients in a blender.

- Blend until smooth.

- Pour into a glass and enjoy!

Prep Time: 5 minutes
Cook Time: 0 minutes
Servings: 1

8. Mocha Milkshake

Ingredients:

- 2 cups coffee ice cream

- 1 cup milk

- 2 tbsp chocolate syrup

Directions:

- Place all ingredients in a blender.

- Blend until smooth.

- Pour into a glass and enjoy!

Prep Time: 5 minutes
Cook Time: 0 minutes
Servings: 1

9. Caramel Milkshake

Ingredients:

- 2 cups vanilla ice cream

- 1 cup milk

- 2 tbsp caramel sauce

Directions:

- Place all ingredients in a blender.

- Blend until smooth.

- Pour into a glass and enjoy!

Prep Time: 5 minutes
Cook Time: 0 minutes
Servings: 1

10. Blueberry Milkshake

Ingredients:

- 2 cups vanilla ice cream

- 1 cup milk

- 1/2 cup fresh blueberries

Directions:

- Place all ingredients in a blender.

- Blend until smooth.

- Pour into a glass and enjoy!

Prep Time: 5 minutes
Cook Time: 0 minutes
Servings: 1

11. Nutella Milkshake

Ingredients:

- 2 cups vanilla ice cream

- 1 cup milk

- 2 tbsp Nutella

Directions:

- Place all ingredients in a blender.

- Blend until smooth.

- Pour into a glass and enjoy!

Prep Time: 5 minutes
Cook Time: 0 minutes
Servings: 1

12. Coconut Milkshake

Ingredients:

- 2 cups coconut ice cream

- 1 cup coconut milk

- 1 tbsp shredded coconut

Directions:

- Place all ingredients in a blender.

- Blend until smooth.

- Pour into a glass and enjoy!

Prep Time: 5 minutes
Cook Time: 0 minutes
Servings: 1

13. Raspberry Milkshake

Ingredients:

- 2 cups vanilla ice cream

- 1 cup milk

- 1/2 cup fresh raspberries

Directions:

- Place all ingredients in a blender.

- Blend until smooth.

- Pour into a glass and enjoy!

Prep Time: 5 minutes
Cook Time: 0 minutes
Servings: 1

14. Pineapple Milkshake

Ingredients:

- 2 cups vanilla ice cream

- 1 cup pineapple juice

- 1/2 cup pineapple chunks

Directions:

- Place all ingredients in a blender.

- Blend until smooth.

- Pour into a glass and enjoy!

Prep Time: 5 minutes
Cook Time: 0 minutes
Servings: 1

15. S'mores Milkshake

Ingredients:

- 2 cups vanilla ice cream

- 1 cup milk

- 2 tbsp chocolate syrup

- 2 graham crackers, crushed

- 1/4 cup mini marshmallows

Directions:

- Place ice cream, milk, and chocolate syrup in a blender.
- Blend until smooth.
- Pour into a glass and top with crushed graham crackers and mini marshmallows.

Prep Time: 5 minutes
Cook Time: 0 minutes
Servings: 1

16. Cherry Vanilla Milkshake

Ingredients:

- 2 cups vanilla ice cream
- 1 cup milk
- 1/2 cup pitted cherries

Directions:

- Place all ingredients in a blender.

- Blend until smooth.

- Pour into a glass and enjoy!

Prep Time: 5 minutes
Cook Time: 0 minutes
Servings: 1

17. Pumpkin Spice Milkshake

Ingredients:

- 2 cups vanilla ice cream

- 1 cup milk

- 1/2 cup pumpkin puree

- 1/2 tsp pumpkin pie spice

Directions:

- Place all ingredients in a blender.

- Blend until smooth.

- Pour into a glass and enjoy!

Prep Time: 5 minutes
Servings: 1

18. Almond Joy Milkshake

Ingredients:

- 2 cups coconut ice cream

- 1 cup almond milk

- 2 tbsp chocolate syrup

- 1 tbsp shredded coconut

Directions:

- Place all ingredients in a blender.

- Blend until smooth.

- Pour into a glass and enjoy!

Prep Time: 5 minutes
Cook Time: 0 minutes
Servings: 1

19. Lemon Cheesecake Milkshake

Ingredients:

- 2 cups vanilla ice cream

- 1 cup milk

- 1/2 cup lemon curd

- 1/4 cup cream cheese

Directions:

- Place all ingredients in a blender.

- Blend until smooth.

- Pour into a glass and enjoy!

Prep Time: 5 minutes
Cook Time: 0 minutes
Servings: 1

20. Salted Caramel Pretzel Milkshake

Ingredients:

- 2 cups vanilla ice cream

- 1 cup milk

- 2 tbsp caramel sauce

- 1/4 cup crushed pretzels

Directions:

- Place ice cream, milk, and caramel sauce in a blender.

- Blend until smooth.

- Pour into a glass and top with crushed pretzels.

Prep Time: 5 minutes
Cook Time: 0 minutes
Servings: 1

Enjoy these delightful milkshakes!

Chapter 9

Troubleshooting and FAQ

Troubleshooting

1. My ice cream isn't as creamy as I expected. What can I do?

Solution: Ensure that you are using full-fat ingredients like whole milk or heavy cream. Low-fat or non-dairy alternatives can result in a less creamy texture. Also, make sure your ingredients are fully blended before freezing.

2. The machine isn't blending the mixture properly.

Solution: Check if the bowl is properly seated and the lid is securely closed. If the mixture is too thick, try adding a small amount of liquid to help it blend more smoothly.

3. My sorbet is too icy.

Solution: Sorbets can become icy if they contain too much water. Adjust the recipe by adding more fruit or using a fruit puree to create a smoother texture. Adding a small amount of sugar or honey can also help to improve the texture.

4. The ice cream mixture is not freezing properly.

Solution: Make sure your freezer is set to the correct temperature (0°F or -18°C). Additionally, check that the mixture was chilled for at least 24 hours before processing.

5. The milkshake is too thin or too thick.

Solution: For a thicker milkshake, use less milk or add more ice cream. For a thinner milkshake, add more milk. Adjust until you reach your desired consistency.

6. The Creamiccino has an uneven texture.

Solution: Ensure that all ingredients are well-mixed before blending. Using pre-chilled ingredients can also help achieve a smoother consistency.

7. The machine is making a loud noise.

Solution: Loud noises can indicate that the machine is overworked. Check that the bowl is not overfilled and that there are no large ice chunks. If necessary, pause the machine and allow it to rest before continuing.

8. My meal replacement shake doesn't taste good.

Solution: Experiment with different flavor combinations and add-ins like fresh fruit, spices, or sweeteners to enhance the taste. Make sure all ingredients are fresh and properly measured.

FAQ

1. Can I use non-dairy milk alternatives in the recipes?

Answer: Yes, you can use non-dairy milk alternatives like almond milk, soy milk, or coconut milk. However, the texture may vary, and non-dairy options may result in a less creamy consistency.

2. How long should I freeze the mixture before processing?

Answer: It's recommended to freeze the mixture for at least 24 hours to ensure it is completely frozen and ready for processing.

3. Can I add mix-ins like chocolate chips or nuts?

Answer: Absolutely! You can add mix-ins like chocolate chips, nuts, or fruit pieces. Add them after the initial blending process and fold them in by hand or use the mix-in setting on your machine.

4. How do I clean the machine?

Answer: Most parts of the Ninja Creami are dishwasher-safe. Consult the user manual for specific cleaning instructions. Ensure all parts are completely dry before reassembling.

5. Can I make sugar-free recipes?

Answer: Yes, you can make sugar-free recipes by using sugar substitutes like stevia, erythritol, or monk fruit sweetener. Adjust the quantity based on your taste preference.

6. My smoothie is separating. How can I fix this?

Answer: Smoothies can separate if they sit for too long. To fix this, simply blend again before drinking. Adding a banana or yogurt can also help to stabilize the mixture.

7. What can I do if my mixture is too sweet or not sweet enough?

Answer: Adjust the sweetness by adding more sweetener if it's not sweet enough, or by diluting with more milk or cream if it's too sweet. Taste your mixture before freezing and adjust as needed.

8. How can I make my recipes healthier?

Answer: Use natural sweeteners like honey or maple syrup, incorporate fruits and vegetables, and opt for low-fat or non-dairy milk alternatives. You can also add protein powder or other nutritional supplements to enhance the health benefits.

9. Can I make recipes ahead of time?

Answer: Yes, you can prepare mixtures ahead of time and store them in the freezer. Just make sure they are in an airtight container to prevent freezer burn.

10. Why is my sorbet too hard to scoop?

Answer: Sorbets can become very hard in the freezer. Let it sit at room temperature for a few minutes before scooping. Adding a small amount of alcohol (like vodka) to the mixture before freezing can also help keep it softer.

Gelato FAQ

1. What is gelato?

Gelato is an Italian-style ice cream known for its rich flavor and smooth texture. It is made with milk, sugar, and flavorings, and often contains less fat and less air compared to traditional ice cream.

2. How is gelato different from ice cream?

Gelato typically has less fat and less air than ice cream, making it denser and creamier. It is also served at a slightly warmer temperature, which enhances its flavor and smooth texture.

3. What ingredients are used to make gelato?

Common ingredients include milk, cream, sugar, and various flavorings like fruits, nuts, chocolate, and coffee. Some gelato recipes also use eggs, but this is less common than in traditional ice cream.

4. Can I make gelato at home without an ice cream maker?

Yes, you can make gelato at home without an ice cream maker by using a blender or food processor and freezing the mixture. However, an ice cream maker helps achieve the best texture by churning the gelato while it freezes.

5. How should gelato be stored?

Gelato should be stored in an airtight container in the freezer. To maintain its creamy texture, let it sit at room temperature for a few minutes before serving.

6. What are some popular gelato flavors?

Popular gelato flavors include vanilla, chocolate, pistachio, hazelnut, stracciatella (chocolate chip), lemon, strawberry, and coffee.

7. Is gelato healthier than ice cream?

Gelato often contains fewer calories and less fat than traditional ice cream, making it a slightly healthier option. However, it still contains sugar and should be enjoyed in moderation.

8. What makes authentic Italian gelato unique?

Authentic Italian gelato is made with fresh, high-quality ingredients and is churned more slowly than ice cream, resulting in a denser, smoother texture. It is also served at a warmer temperature, which enhances its flavor.

9. Can gelato be made with non-dairy milk?

Yes, gelato can be made with non-dairy milk such as almond milk, coconut milk, or soy milk. These alternatives can create delicious gelato that is suitable for those with lactose intolerance or a vegan diet.

10. How long does homemade gelato last?

Homemade gelato is best enjoyed within a week of making it, but it can be stored in the freezer for up to a month. After that, the texture and flavor may start to degrade.

11. Why is my gelato too hard or icy?

Gelato can become too hard or icy if it contains too much water or is stored at too low a temperature. To improve the texture, make sure to use the right balance of ingredients and let the gelato soften slightly at room temperature before serving.

12. Can gelato be used in desserts other than a scoop in a cone or cup?

Yes, gelato can be used in a variety of desserts, such as gelato sandwiches, affogato (gelato with espresso poured over it), gelato cakes, and even as a topping for pies and cakes.

13. What is the best way to serve gelato?

Gelato is best served slightly softened, so let it sit at room temperature for a few minutes before scooping. Use a warmed gelato scoop to make serving easier and create smooth, round scoops.

14. Are there any special tools needed to make gelato at home?

While an ice cream maker helps achieve the best texture, you can make gelato with a blender or food processor. A good gelato scoop and airtight storage containers are also useful.

15. Can I add mix-ins to gelato?

Yes, you can add mix-ins like chocolate chips, nuts, or fruit pieces to gelato. Add them towards the end of the churning process to evenly distribute the mix-ins without over-churning the gelato.

16. How can I make gelato with a smooth and creamy texture?

To achieve a smooth and creamy texture, use high-quality ingredients, chill the mixture before churning, and avoid over-churning. An ice cream maker can help, but you can also blend the mixture well and stir it periodically while freezing.

17. Why does gelato melt faster than ice cream?

Gelato melts faster because it is typically served at a warmer temperature than ice cream and contains less fat. The lower fat content and denser texture contribute to its faster melting rate.

18. Is gelato gluten-free?

Many gelato flavors are naturally gluten-free, but it's important to check the ingredients, especially for flavors that may contain cookies, brownies, or other gluten-containing mix-ins. Always ask if you're unsure.

19. Can I make sugar-free gelato?

Yes, you can make sugar-free gelato using sugar substitutes like stevia, erythritol, or monk fruit sweetener. Keep in mind that the texture and sweetness may differ from traditional gelato.

20. What is the origin of gelato?

Gelato originated in Italy and has been enjoyed there for centuries. It became popular worldwide for its rich flavor and creamy texture, with many regions in Italy known for their unique gelato-making traditions and flavors.

By following these troubleshooting tips and FAQs, you can ensure your Ninja Creami Deluxe recipes turn out perfectly every time. Enjoy experimenting with different flavors and textures to create your perfect frozen treats.

Conclusion

Congratulations on reaching the end of "The Ninja Creami Deluxe Cookbook: 140 Easy Recipes for Homemade Sorbet, Gelato, Ice Cream, Milkshakes, Creamiccino, Smoothie, and Meal Replacement Shakes for Beginners and Experts." You've embarked on a delicious journey, discovering the endless possibilities that your Ninja Creami has to offer.

By now, you've likely experimented with a variety of recipes, from creamy ice creams and refreshing sorbets to thick milkshakes and nutritious meal replacement shakes. Each recipe was designed to be simple, allowing you to create delightful treats with ease, no matter your skill level.

The Ninja Creami isn't just a kitchen appliance; it's a gateway to creativity and healthier eating. You've learned how to make desserts and drinks that are not only tasty but also tailored to your dietary needs and preferences. Whether you're indulging in a rich, chocolate ice cream or enjoying a vibrant, fruit-packed smoothie, you've made choices that satisfy your cravings and nourish your body.

We hope this cookbook has inspired you to continue exploring new flavors and techniques. Keep experimenting, adjust the recipes to your taste, and don't be afraid to try something new. The joy of homemade treats lies in the freedom to create exactly what you love.

Thank you for choosing this cookbook and allowing us to be a part of your culinary adventure. We hope it has brought joy, flavor, and a bit of fun to your kitchen. Remember, the best recipes are the ones made with love and shared with others. Happy creating, and may your Ninja Creami continue to bring you delicious moments for years to come.

About the Author

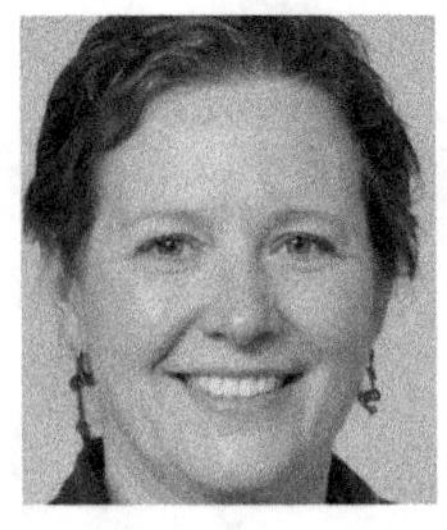

Fredia S. Prather, author of The Ninja Creami Deluxe Cookbook, is a culinary enthusiast and accomplished author. Her expertise in blending flavors and crafting innovative recipes has made her a respected figure in the culinary world. Prather's cookbook offers delicious and creative ways to utilize the Ninja Creami, showcasing her passion for food and cooking.

www.ingramcontent.com/pod-product-compliance
Lightning Source LLC
Chambersburg PA
CBHW051557250726